MW01599642

THIS JOURNAL BELONGS TO:

....

....

A OWN notebooks PRODUCTION

Manufactured by Amazon.ca
Acheson, AB

11694444R00066